I0703697

Table of Contents

With a chair, you can go places in some of your favorite poses that you have yet been unable to go! This article offers a new approach to some of your favorite poses. You may have seen the row of chairs in the back of your local yoga studio and wondered, Why have I never used one of those? Or maybe you thought using a chair - or any prop - is only for people who have trouble achieving the "full pose." Not at all.

It is true that chairs can be used to make poses more accessible to those with mobility issues. A chair is sometimes used to access a feeling of release and relaxation. But you may not know that a chair can also be a surprisingly empowering way to gain a deeper understanding of your alignment, and increase your focus, flexibility, and strength. With a chair, you can go places in some of your favorite poses that you have yet been unable to go!

In this guide book you will be exposed to few popular yoga poses you might already be working on that can be augmented by adding in this simple prop. Chair yoga is an adapted yoga practice that allows you to stay seated while practicing yoga focused poses. It can be practiced by anyone who wants to enjoy the benefits of yoga and may (or may not) have mobility limitations.

For example, chair yoga is great for anyone who needs more support, is managing an injury, or wants a more therapeutic approach to the practice. Chair yoga is an accessible form of yoga to be enjoyed by anyone, no matter their body type, limitations, or abilities. Chair yoga is a promising form of exercise for older adults.

It may help people with certain health conditions, such as arthritis, to exercise without putting pressure on joints. It may also reduce the fear of falling, and help people who are not used to exercise to begin improving their strength and balance. In addition to improving physical health, yoga also involves mindfulness, which can benefit mental health and well-being.

Older adults who are new to chair yoga may benefit from speaking with a health professional for advice on how to try it safely. Read on to learn more about chair yoga for seniors, including whether it works, the benefits, and some poses to try.

UNDERSTANDING CHAIR YOGA POSES

We tend to think of yoga as an athletic endeavor that has to be done on a mat. Yoga practice is about much more than the physical [poses]; the practice includes skills like breathing, regulating your emotions, and practicing self-care.

Meaning of Chair Yoga

Chair yoga, a gentle form of yoga that's done while seated or using a chair for balance, makes the practice more accessible. In chair yoga, it's possible to move into poses like cat/cow, warrior, sun salutations and forward folds, all while seated. Start where you are, use what you have, do what you can," is perfect for chair yoga. You're there to work and to challenge yourself, but it's about knowing what's right for you.

I think of yoga poses as adaptable to a student's body and not the other way around. Whether yoga is done in a chair or on the mat, the practice still focuses on the same core principles: focusing on your breath, paying attention to your thoughts, and staying in the moment.

The Benefits of Chair Yoga

Research shows yoga is linked to decreased levels of stress, anxiety, and depression, lowered cholesterol and blood pressure, improved energy, better sleep quality, less pain, and reduced body mass index. Chair yoga is also a good, safe workout for Beginners. It's a great way to work your core, explore the different range of motion of the joints and prioritize movement.

When you're sitting down or using a chair for balance, the safety factor goes way up. Practicing yoga while seated benefits those who are limited in their ability to perform movements without stability and support. Chair yoga classes are widely available in senior centers and retirement communities, as older adults are its biggest target audience.

People who fall in the obesity category and people with neurological diseases are also good candidates for chair yoga. Office workers can also take advantage of chair yoga's adaptations to do stretches at work. In general, yoga can help manage stress and symptoms of depression and relieve anxiety. It can also boost your mood and quality of sleep.

These beneficial effects may be especially important for those bound to a chair or less able to perform other types of exercise.

Chair Yoga Sequence

Because chair yoga is all about adaptability, it should come as no surprise that the particular chair you use is not important; you don't have to run out and buy a specialized yoga chair. That said, chairs with wheels are not ideal (unless you can lock the wheels to keep the chair from moving). If your feet do not reach the floor, you put blocks or a folded yoga mat under your feet to give yourself a firm foundation.

Who Should Try Chair Yoga?

Although chair yoga is often promoted as a practice for those who may struggle with a mat practice, anyone can benefit from this type of gentle exercise.

Tips for Working out When You're Over 50

Chair yoga is particularly well-suited to people who use wheelchairs and those rehabilitating after surgeries, living with chronic illnesses, or dealing with balance issues that make it hard to get down onto a yoga mat. It's also perfect for a quick workout during the workday or while traveling. It's not about the outcome. It's not about striking the perfect pose.

Whether yoga is taught on the mat or in a chair, it's all about being healthy. Chair yoga is also ideal for beginners who might be intimidated by a traditional mat practice because it offers a safe way to learn the poses, Minard adds.

Where to Find Chair Yoga Classes

You can find chair yoga classes at community centers, fitness facilities, and yoga studios. There are also a lot of online options. In this video, Kelly provides detailed instructions for a short chair yoga practice that is suitable for all levels.

How to Get Started

To practice at home, use a sturdy chair (an office chair on wheels or overstuffed armchair are not appropriate for chair yoga). chair that naturally positions your hips slightly higher than your knees and allows you to put both feet flat on the floor. If your feet aren't flat on the ground, your weight is all in your spine and if the chair is too low and your knees are above your hips, there is more impingement on your hips.

You want to be able to do slow, controlled movements without putting extra stress on your back or hips. Make sure the chair is on a stable surface like carpet or a yoga mat to keep it from slipping. You can also position the back of the chair against a wall for extra stability. Yoga props like blocks, straps, and resistance bands that are common in mat practices aren't required for chair yoga -- unless you want an extra challenge.

Chair yoga is a good starting point to use muscles you haven't used in a while without the potential risks of overloading [your muscles and joints] or falling. If the resistance from your body weight isn't enough of a challenge, you can add light hand weights, ankle weights or resistance bands to your chair yoga practice.

11 Chair Yoga Poses You Can Do at Home

Seated yoga has many benefits and it's easy to practice in your own space. Chair yoga is a general term for practices that modify yoga poses so they can be done while seated in a chair. These modifications make yoga accessible to people who cannot stand, lack the mobility to move easily from standing to seated to supine positions, or want a quick break from office work.

Many of the basic body mechanics of the individual postures remain the same. Just like with traditional mat yoga, chair yoga moves include versions of twists, hip stretches, forward bends, and mild backends. In addition to a good stretch, chair yoga participants can also enjoy other health benefits of yoga.2 This can include improved muscle tone, better breathing habits, stress reduction, better sleep, and an improved sense of well-being.

These eleven adapted yoga poses may seem familiar if you have practiced traditional yoga. You can perform them as a sequence or choose a few to string together into a flow that suits your available time and ability. Remember to follow the breathing techniques and be mindful of your posture as you move through them.

1. Chair Cat-Cow Stretch

- ✓ Sit on a chair with the spine long and both feet on the floor. Place your hands on your knees or the tops of your thighs.
- ✓ On an inhale, arch your spine and roll your shoulders down and back, bringing your shoulder blades onto your back. This is cow position.
- ✓ On an exhale, round your spine and drop your chin to your chest, letting the shoulder and head come forward. This is cat position.

✓ Continue moving between cow on the inhalations and cat on the exhalations for five breaths.

2. Chair Raised Hands Pose - Urdhva Hastasana

✓ On an inhalation, raise your arms toward the ceiling.

✓ Maintain good upper body posture with the shoulders relaxed and rib cage sitting naturally over the hips. Anchor your sit bones in your chair seat and reach up from there.

3. Chair Forward Bend - Uttanasana

✓ On an exhalation, come into a forward bend over the legs. Let the hands rest on the floor if they reach it. Let the head hang heavy.

✓ On an inhalation, raise the arms back up over the head. Repeat this movement between a raised arms position and a forward fold several times, moving with the breath.

4. Chair Extended Side Angle - Utthita Parsvakonasana

- ✓ After your final forward bend, stay folded. Bring your left fingertips to the floor on the outside of your left foot. If your left hand doesn't come easily to the floor, place a block under it or bring it to your left knee instead and twist from there.

- ✓ Open your chest as you twist to the right on an inhale, bringing your right arm and gaze up at the ceiling. This is your chair version of extended side angle pose. Hold here for several breaths. Bring the right arm down on an exhale.

- ✓ Do the same position with the right arm down and the left arm up.

5. Chair Pigeon - Eka Pada Rajakapotasana

- ✓ Come back up to sit. Bring your right ankle to rest on your left thigh, keeping the knee in line with your ankle as much as possible. Hold this chair pigeon for three to five breaths.
- ✓ You may forward bend to intensify the stretch if you like. Repeat with the left leg.

6. Chair Eagle - Garudasana

- ✓ Cross your right thigh over your left thigh for eagle pose. If you can, wrap the right foot all the way around the left calf.
- ✓ Cross your left arm over the right one at the elbow. Bend the elbows and bring your palms to touch.
- ✓ Lift the elbows while dropping the shoulders away from the ears. Hold three to five breaths.
- ✓ Repeat on the other side.

7. Chair Spinal Twist - Ardha Matsyendrasana

- ✓ Come to sit sideways on the chair, facing to the left. Twist your torso toward the left, holding onto the back of the chair, for a spinal twist.
- ✓ Lengthen your spine on each inhale and twist on each exhale for five breaths.
- ✓ Move your legs around to the right side of the chair and repeat the twist to the right side.

8. Chair Warrior I - Virabhadrasana I

- ✓ Now keep the right leg in position over the side of the chair while you swing the left leg behind you.
- ✓ Plant the sole of the left foot on the floor roughly parallel to the seat of the chair and straighten the left leg.
- ✓ Keep your torso facing over the right leg as you raise your arms up to the ceiling on a

inhale coming to warrior I. Hold for three breaths.

9. Chair Warrior II - Virabhadrasana II

- ✓ On an exhale, open up the arms with the right arm coming forward and the left arm going back.
- ✓ Draw the left hip back and turn the torso to the left, so that it is aligned with the front of the chair.
- ✓ Gaze out over the right fingertips and hold warrior II for three breaths.

10. Reverse Warrior

- ✓ Let the left arm come down the left leg and lift the right arm up to the ceiling on an inhale for reverse warrior. Hold for three breaths.
- ✓ Bring both legs to the front of the chair before coming to sit sideways on the chair

facing left and going through the series of three warrior poses on the left side.

11. Final Relaxation: Chair Savasana

Take a few minutes to sit with your eyes closed and hands in your lap at the end of your practice. This seated savasana will help your body absorb all the good effects of the poses you have done and transition you into the rest of your day.

Chair yoga, a modified version of vinyasa yoga, is an accessible exercise option for anyone with reduced mobility or who's short on time. If you've found yourself living a more sedentary life due to COVID or you're simply bent over a computer screen for most of your waking hours, you might be looking for more ways to get active. But busy schedules mean it might feel impossible to find time to take a break and center yourself.

Chair yoga is exactly what it sounds like: Yoga in, or with the assistance of, a chair. It uses various modified poses from the widely-practiced vinyasa style, coupled with meditative breathing, to help you get a relaxing, de-stressing stretch.

What Is Chair Yoga?

There are two main types of chair yoga. "One where the student or practitioner uses the chair as a prop. For example, there are modifications to different postures, where the person might stand up and lean on the chair or put one of their legs resting on the chair. The other is the kind of yoga I teach to seniors in assisted living, [which is] 100 percent seated.

If the target audience is severely limited in mobility, they can still do a really meaningful practice of yoga, particularly because the foundation of all practice is the breath. Chair yoga—and yoga in general—is for everyone, no matter what their skill level may be. Anyone can benefit from [chair yoga], but particularly folks who are at their desks the majority of the day [or] people who spend a lot of time on their feet.

This is a great way to practice yoga without asking for a lot from you physically. Though our idea of yoga may be centered on the physical aspect of the poses, what differentiates the practice from simply stretching is the focus on managing the breath. '"Yoga teaches you to use the breath. That's what's really benefiting the body.

You'll notice that in any type of yoga class that you take, you're being guided back to your breath. A lot of times we forget that we can always come back to the breath when we're feeling overwhelmed or tension in the body. Practicing deep breathing really helps to relax the body. The stretching is just an additional benefit.

yoga expert for nine years recommends focusing on your breathing before you get started. "[You] can sit in a chair and tune in to your breathing," he says. "That's really important. Tune in. Am I breathing shallowly? Am I only allowing a certain amount of myself to be oxygenated? Can I let in more?"

Forward Bend

The first pose you can try—especially if the morning has been stressful—is a forward bend. According to Brown, this is a modification of the standing forward fold. Bend forward, hinging from your hips, and reach your hands towards the floor. "Your hands don't have to go all the way to the floor," Brown noted. "But, you do want your head to hang heavy. Your hands can stop wherever they want to stop.

You can rest your hands on your shins. The most important thing here is that the neck is relaxed. The forward bend is helpful for those of us who slouch, as it counterbalances the hunched position. It is also instrumental in managing anxious feelings and thoughts. This helps with anxiety. When you're experiencing anxiety, your heart is racing; you're having a hard time catching your breath.

When you place your head between your knees, that helps to relax the system and helps you regulate your breathing.

Spinal Twist

Another exercise you can try is the spinal twist, which both Jacobson and Brown suggest. Keep your feet planted on the floor and gently twist to one side, bringing your arms around the back of your chair. You want to inhale at the center and exhale during the twist. It's meant to be a gentle opening of the spine, so don't push the pose past what is comfortable.

And it's perfectly fine if you hear some pops. "That's something that naturally happens in the twisting poses. It's not a bad thing. It's just something that is naturally happening to the spine because we're twisting. I always tell people to honor their bodies. If they're in a twist and it feels too intense, then just come back a little bit closer towards the front.

You don't have to twist all the way back. Just a gentle twist, stopping where it feels good for you.

Seated Cat-Cow

If you've taken an introductory yoga course, you are probably familiar with the cat-cow pose. This can also be done in a chair. Again, plant your feet on the ground and place your hands on your knees. As you inhale (slowly!), open up your chest and arch your back, allowing your gaze to tilt towards the ceiling. On the exhale, round your spine into the cat pose.

Hip Swirl

One last exercise you can do is what Jacobson calls a hip swirl. "You're just circling the hips in one direction, along with the breathing," she says. "Inhaling as you circle those hips forward and exhaling as you circle back. You would do that for three to five breath cycles and then switch direction. The feet are going to stay planted this whole time. The feet are grounding you. Your tailbone is rooted into the chair.

Ten Reasons to Do Chair Yoga

1. Chairs don't take up much floor space.

Many places where I teach do not have the floor space for 10 mats, but most places have space for 10 chairs. You can create an intimate circle, or space chairs out if you have more room and want to do sweeping arm movements.

2. Chairs are easy to come by.

Everybody has one or has access to one. Alternatively, you could use that nearby park bench or low concrete wall. Easy access to a chair removes a barrier to yoga practice. No more "the dog ate my yoga mat" excuses!

3. Chairs are accessible to anyone who can sit.

That includes a lot of people. A surprising number of seemingly able-bodied people who I come across greet me with lots of nervousness until I reassure them they will not be on the floor. People have all sorts of body issues that you may never know about. Somehow, a chair is an equalizer for them.

4. The quality and range of movement one can achieve from sitting in a chair is surprising.

In one of my classes, a veteran marathon runner had sweat beading down her face just from doing a seated cat and cow and lateral movement of the spine in a chair. She simply had not moved her body in this particular way before, and her body was responding. There's no downside; fit people can still "feel good" from the slow movement. Non-fit people - or perhaps folks who are a little disconnected from their bodies – usually can give themselves permission to try something as non-threatening as sitting in a chair.

5. A chair can be a great prop.

You can sit on it. You can stand and use it to help you balance, or put your foot on it for some hip work. If you like the pose Balancing Half Moon but struggle with it, try using a chair instead of blocks. It's a beautiful and freeing thing. The idea is to find steadiness and ease in every pose, which is the very thing that the ancient sage Patanjali wrote in Yoga Sutra 2.46: sthira sukham asanam.

6. Chairs are a great aid to posture.

Sit at the very front of your chair with your feet hip width apart and firmly planted on the floor to challenge your posture. Do this for 15 minutes each day, and see how your posture and your breathing will improve.

7. People in wheelchairs feel special.

They bring their own chairs and love being part of the group and participating just like everyone else is. Normalizing is good.

8. Chairs slow you down.

Some of us need all the help we can get. It is hard to hurt yourself when you slow down. Often, it is harder to move mindfully when we are trying to move slowly. We feel more. But that's the idea: to feel more, physically and mentally, and to notice what's going on internally.

9. Using a chair is humbling. Practicing in one is good for the ego.

There's no pretention here; just you and the chair and maybe a block or two. It is okay to balance with both feet on the floor. Humbleness is good. Neither chairs nor yoga have the corner on the market when it comes to relaxation. There are many ways to practice, relax and meditate. However, if you have never tried yoga, chair yoga is a great way to start.

10. Using a chair allows REAL people to do REAL yoga.

Over the ten years I have been teaching yoga from a chair, I have been able to persuade many a person that "yes, this really is yoga, and no, you do not have to stand on your head or be flexible to practice." That prevailing image folks have in their heads about yoga intimidates many people. Historically, yoga was almost entirely non-posture based, as is evidenced by Patanjali's Yoga Sutra Yogas citta vritti nirodhah," meaning "Yoga is the cessation of the fluctuations of the mind." Yoga originated as meditation practice.

So, why do we continue to be bombarded by images from the yoga "industry" that make us think it is all about the slick arm balance of a super bendy person? Often, these poses are achievable by only a small percentage of people practicing yoga and may even be contraindicated for most people practicing yoga. So, let's be real and honest.

I am committed to promoting the message that if you can breathe, you can do yoga. Like they say at TED, that's an "idea worth spreading. "I hope you pull up a chair and join me.

When you think of exercise equipment, the first thing that probably comes to mind is a set of dumbbells or a treadmill. And if you have yoga in mind, the image of a mat on the floor is probably what comes to mind. But what if you don't have any of that equipment? Or what if you're not able to get down on the floor? That's where chair yoga comes in!

Chair yoga is a type of yoga that can be done either seated in a chair or standing using a chair for support. This type of yoga is perfect for beginners or anyone who has difficulty getting down on the floor. It's also great for people who are limited in their mobility or are dealing with injuries. Chair yoga is a great way to get started with yoga, and it can be just as effective as traditional yoga.

Meaning of Chair Yoga

Asanas are the foundation of a yoga practice. They are designed to stretch, strengthen, and promote flexibility. However, not all yoga poses are suitable for everyone. People who have difficulty getting up and down from the floor, or who have other physical limitations, may find traditional yoga poses difficult or even impossible to do. Enter chair yoga. Chair yoga is a type of yoga that can be done while seated in a chair, or while standing using a chair for support.

It is an accessible form of yoga that benefits people of all ages and abilities. Unlike traditional yoga, chair yoga does not require you to be super flexible or strong. It is a gentle and low-impact form of exercise that can help improve your overall health and well-being.

Who Can Do Chair Yoga?

This gentle form of yoga is suitable for just about anyone. However, it is especially beneficial for:

- ✓ People with limited mobility: whether due to age, injury, or chronic health conditions
- ✓ People who are new to yoga and want to ease into it gradually
- ✓ Pregnant women
- ✓ People who are looking for a low-impact form of exercise
- ✓ People who live sedentary lifestyles and want to add more movement into their day

Benefit of Chair Yoga Work

The benefits of traditional yoga are well-documented. Luckily for those who cannot do traditional yoga, chair yoga has many of the same benefits. Some of the potential benefits of chair yoga include:

Increased Flexibility

The ability to bend, twist, and stretch is important, not just for yoga but for daily life as well. When you do chair yoga regularly, you may find that your range of motion gradually increases. This can make it easier to do activities like reaching for items on a high shelf or putting on your socks in the morning. With time, your range of motion may improve such that you can perform traditional yoga poses.

Improved Strength

Chair yoga can help improve your overall strength, including the muscles in your arms, legs, and core. It does this by using your body weight as resistance. As you get stronger, you may find it easier to do everyday activities like carrying groceries or getting in and out of a car. Plus, stronger muscles can help protect your joints from injuries.

Better Balance

Yoga, in general, can help improve your balance. While you may not be doing standing balance poses in chair yoga, the asanas can still help you develop better balance. They improve your mind-body connection and help you learn to control your body while in different positions. This can come in handy if you ever find yourself off-balance, such as when you trip on a curb.

Relaxation

One of the main goals of yoga is to promote relaxation. Chair yoga is no different. The slow, controlled movements and deep breathing can help you clear your mind and ease tension in your body. This can lead to improved sleep, reduced stress levels, and a general sense of well-being.

Types of Chair Yoga Poses

There are many different types of chair yoga poses. Some poses can be done while seated in a chair while others require you to stand using the chair for support. Here are a few examples of common chair yoga poses:

Chair Yoga Sun Salutation

This pose is a series of movements that are often done at the beginning of a traditional yoga practice. They help warm up your body and get your blood flowing. To do the chair yoga sun salutation:

- ✓ Sit up tall in your chair with your feet flat on the ground.
- ✓ Inhale and reach your arms up overhead.
- ✓ Exhale and fold forward, placing your hands on your knees.
- ✓ Inhale and lift your head, shoulders, and chest.
- ✓ Exhale and round your back.
- ✓ Inhale and reach your arms up overhead again.
- ✓ Exhale and return to the starting position.

✓ Repeat this sequence for 10–20 breaths.

Seated Mountain Pose

This pose is a good way to start your chair yoga practice. It helps you focus on your breath and connect with your body. To perform the seated mountain pose:

- ✓ Sit up tall in your chair with your feet flat on the ground.
- ✓ Relax your shoulders and lengthen your spine.
- ✓ Take a few deep breaths and focus on your breath.

Seated Cat-Cow Pose

This pose targets your spine. Spinal twists are important for improving flexibility and range of motion in your back. To do the seated cat-cow pose:

- ✓ Sit up tall in your chair with your feet flat on the floor.
- ✓ Place your hands on your knees.
- ✓ As you inhale, arch your back and look up.
- ✓ As you exhale, round your back and look down.
- ✓ Repeat this movement for 10–20 breaths.°0
- ✓ Seated Forward Bend: This pose stretches your back, shoulders, and hamstrings. It's also a good pose for calming the nervous system. To do the seated forward bend:
- ✓ Sit up tall in your chair with your feet flat on the ground.
- ✓ Inhale and reach your arms up overhead.
- ✓ Exhale and fold forward, placing your hands on your knees.
- ✓ Relax your head and neck.
- ✓ Hold this position for 5–10 breaths.

Seated Twist

This pose stretches your back and shoulders. It also helps improve digestion. To do the seated twist:

- ✓ Sit up tall in your chair with your feet flat on the ground.
- ✓ Place your right hand on your left knee and your left hand behind you on the chair.
- ✓ Inhale and lengthen your spine.
- ✓ Exhale and twist to the left, looking over your left shoulder.
- ✓ Hold this position for 5–10 breaths.
- ✓ Repeat on the other side.

Supported Bridge Pose

This pose stretches your chest, neck, and back. It also helps improve posture. To do the supported bridge pose:

- ✓ Sit up straight with your back against the back of the chair.

✓ Place your feet flat on the ground and hip-width apart.

✓ Place your hands on your knees.

✓ Inhale and lift your hips, tilting your pelvis forward.

✓ Exhale and arch your back.

✓ Hold this position for 5–10 breaths.

How Often Should You Do Chair Yoga?

Chair yoga is a gentle form of exercise that can be done daily. If you're just starting, you may want to practice chair yoga 3–4 times per week. That's because your muscles will need time to adjust to the new movements and positions. As your body becomes stronger and more flexible, you can increase the frequency of your practice.

How Long Will It Take To See Results?

That depends on your goals. If you're looking to improve your flexibility, you may see results within a few weeks. If you're trying to build muscle strength, it may take a few months to see significant results. However, you'll likely feel the benefits of chair yoga after your very first session. That's because physical activity often has the immediate effect of improving mood and energy levels.

So even if you don't see major changes in your body right away, know that chair yoga is still working its magic!

Should You Feel Sore After Chair Yoga?

Soreness is normal after any type of physical activity, including chair yoga. However, the soreness should go away after a day or two. If you're feeling pain that lasts longer than that, it's important to listen to your body and take a break from yoga.

How Can Beginners Get Started with Chair Yoga?

Beginners should follow these tips to get started with chair yoga:

Start slow: Don't try to do too much too soon. Begin with just a few poses and gradually add more.

Listen to your body: If a pose feels uncomfortable, stop doing it. And if you're feeling pain, take a break.

Breathe: Don't forget to breathe! Breath is an important part of yoga.

Find a comfortable seat: A sturdy, comfortable chair is essential for chair yoga. Make sure the chair is at a height that allows your feet to touch the ground.

Practice regularly: The more you do chair yoga, the better the results. Try to practice 3–4 times per week.

Warm-up and cool-down: Before you start your yoga practice, take a few minutes to warm up with some basic stretches. And when you're finished, do some gentle stretches to cool down.

Combine it with other activities: Chair yoga is a great way to add movement to your day. But it's not the only way. Combine chair yoga with other activities like walking, swimming, or Tai Chi to get the most benefit.

Chair Yoga on The BetterMe App

Starting out on your own can be daunting, and going to regular yoga classes isn't always possible. That's where the BetterMe app comes in to make things easier for you. The chair yoga section has a series of easy-to-follow routines that target different areas. Pick the ones you like or need the most and add them to your daily routine. Watch the instructional videos to make sure you're doing the poses correctly.

With gentle warm-up and cool-down stretches included, these workout sessions can easily become a part of your day. Choose between different durations and difficulty levels to find a routine that suits you.

YOGA POSES YOU CAN DO IN A CHAIR

It's popular these days to say "yoga is for everybody." But is that really true? Can it really be practiced by everyone? Even those who, due to age, inflexibility, or injury, need to practice completely from a chair? Absolutely! In fact, seniors may be able to get more out of yoga than most students. Since the brain's two hemispheres are used more equally as we age, we can bring a better overall awareness to yoga, thus utilizing the mind-body connection more effectively than younger students.

Keep in mind that many seniors who are physically fit have no limitations when it comes to practicing yoga, except maybe using the adaptation devices many younger people use as well, such as blocks or straps. However, chair yoga may be the way to go for people:

✓ With balance issues

✓ Looking to start slowly

✓ Who would just feel more confident starting out this way

It not only has the benefits of regular yoga, such as helping with stress, pain, and fatigue — but it can also help with joint lubrication, balance, and even age-specific issues like menopause and arthritis. This sequence will benefit anyone who prefers to do yoga in a chair, such as seniors or those in a chair at work. Keep in mind that you want a sturdy chair that you feel comfortable and stable in.

That means no office chairs with wheels or anything that feels rickety. And be sure to start off each new pose by making sure your butt is planted firmly in the seat. You will want to sit toward the front edge of the seat but still on the seat enough to feel stable.

Seated Mountain (Tadasana)

This is a great pose to simply engage your core, check in with your posture, and focus on your breath. Come to this pose after each of the poses below.

- ✓ Take a deep breath and sit up straight, extending your spine.
- ✓ As you exhale, root down into the chair with your sit bones (the lowest part of your tailbone, or the two points that take the weight when you sit).
- ✓ Your legs should be at 90-degree angles, knees directly over your ankles.
- ✓ You want to have a little room between your knees.
- ✓ Typically, your fist should fit between your knees, though your skeletal structure may require more room than this.
- ✓ Take a deep breath and as you exhale, roll your shoulders down your back, pull your

bellybutton in toward your spine, and relax your arms down at your sides.

✓ If your chair has armrests, you may need to have them out to the front just a little or a bit wider, to clear the armrests.

✓ Engage your legs by lifting your toes and pressing firmly into all four corners of your feet.

Warrior I (Virbhadrasana I)

✓ Starting in Seated Mountain, take a deep breath. As you inhale, lift your arms out to the sides, then raise your hands up to meet above your head.

✓ Lace your fingers together, keeping your pointer fingers and thumbs out, so you're pointing at the ceiling directly over your head.

✓ As you exhale, roll your shoulders away from your ears, letting your shoulder blades slide down your back. This will engage the shoulder capsule (the muscles that hold your shoulder joint together).

✓ Continue to take deep and even breaths as you settle in here, taking at least 5 deep breaths before you release your clasped hands on an exhale and let your arms gently float back to your sides.

✓ Seated Forward Bend (Paschimottanasana)

✓ Inhale in Seated Mountain, focusing on extending your spine, and simply fold over your legs.

✓ You can start with your hands resting on your thighs and slide them down your legs as you fold for a little extra support, or you can keep them at your sides as you work toward laying your torso on your thighs.

✓ Take 5 or more even breaths in this pose. It massages your intestines, helping with digestion, as well as passively lengthening your spine and stretching your back muscles.

✓ When ready, inhale as you lift your torso back to an upright position.

Eagle Arms (Garudasana Arms)

This pose relaxes your shoulders and upper back as it stabilizes and flexes your shoulder joint.

✓ Take a breath and then, as you inhale, stretch your arms out to your sides.

✓ As you exhale, bring them in front of you, swinging your right arm under your left and grabbing your shoulders with the opposite hands, giving yourself a hug.

✓ If you have more flexibility in your shoulders, you can release your grip and continue wrapping your forearms around each other until your right fingers rest in your left palm.

✓ Inhaling, lift your elbows a few inches higher.

✓ Exhaling, roll your shoulders down, relaxing them away from your ears.

✓ Take a few breaths, repeating the elbow lift
and shoulder roll if you like.

Reverse Arm Hold

This stretches your shoulders and opens up your
chest, which can help with posture, stress, and
breathing difficulties.

✓ As you inhale, stretch both arms out to your
sides, palms down.

✓ As you exhale, roll both shoulders forward a
little, which rolls your

✓ palms so they're facing behind you, then
bend your elbows and let your hands

✓ swing behind your back.

✓ Clasp hands in any way you like (fingers,
hands, wrists, or elbows) and

✓ gently pull your hands away from each
other without releasing your hold.

✓ If you gripped a wrist or elbow, note which
side it's on.

✓ After you've taken 5 slow, even breaths with arms clasped this way, reclasp the other wrist or elbow and hold for 5 breaths.

Simple Seated Twist (Parivrtta Sukhasana)

✓ Twisting poses help with lower back pain and aid digestion and circulation. They're often called "detox" poses.

✓ Though you will have your chair back to help you twist here, keep in mind that you don't want to use the chair to yank yourself into a deeper twist.

✓ Your body will have a natural stopping point. Don't force it by pulling with your hands. Forcing a twist can cause serious injury.

✓ As you inhale, extend your spine again and raise your arms out to your sides and up.

✓ As you exhale, gently twist to the right with your upper body and lower your arms —

your right hand will rest on the top of the chair back and help you to gently twist, your left hand will rest at your side.

- ✓ Look over your right shoulder. Use your grip on the chair to help you stay in the twist but not to deepen it.
- ✓ After 5 breaths, release this twist and return to facing the front.
- ✓ Repeat on your left side.

Single-Leg Stretch (Janu Sirsasana)

- ✓ You can inch a little closer to the edge of your seat for this one. Just be sure you're still on the chair enough that you won't slide off.
- ✓ Sitting up tall, stretch your right leg out, resting your heel on the floor, toes pointing up — the closer to the edge of the seat you are, the straighter your leg can get.

- ✓ But again, be mindful of how supported you are before folding forward.
- ✓ Rest both hands on your outstretched leg. As you inhale, raise up through your spine, and as you exhale, begin to bend over your right leg, sliding your hands down your leg as you go.
- ✓ Take this stretch as far as you like while not straining or forcing anything and still feeling supported, both by the chair and by your hands.
- ✓ If you're able to reach lower on your leg, consider grasping the back of your calf or your ankle.
- ✓ Inhale and exhale slowly and evenly 5 times in this position, gently going deeper each time, and then release the pose by using an inhale to help you rise.
- ✓ Repeat this pose with your left leg outstretched, double-checking how supported your body is on the edge of the

chair and realigning your right leg's knee over your ankle before you bend over.

The 10 Best Yoga Poses for Back Pain

- ✓ Cat-Cow
- ✓ Downward-Facing Dog
- ✓ Extended Triangle
- ✓ Sphinx Pose
- ✓ Cobra Pose
- ✓ Locust Pose
- ✓ Bridge Pose
- ✓ Half Lord of the Fishes
- ✓ Two-Knee Spinal Twist
- ✓ Child's Pose

Yoga poses like cat-cow, lotus pose, and triangle pose may help strengthen and relax muscles, which may relieve back pain. If you're dealing with back pain, yoga may be just what the doctor ordered. Yoga is a mind-body therapy that's often recommended to treat not only back pain but the stress that accompanies it. The appropriate poses can relax and strengthen your body.

Practicing yoga for even a few minutes a day can help you gain more awareness of your body. This will help you notice where you're holding tension and where you have imbalances. You can use this awareness to bring yourself into balance and alignment.

1. Cat-Cow

This gentle, accessible backbend stretches and mobilizes the spine. Practicing this pose also stretches your torso, shoulders, and neck.

Muscles worked:

- ✓ Erector Spinae
- ✓ Rectus Abdominis
- ✓ Triceps
- ✓ Serratus Anterior
- ✓ Gluteus Maximus

To do this:

- ✓ Get on all fours.
- ✓ Place your wrists underneath your shoulders and your knees underneath your hips.
- ✓ Balance your weight evenly between all four points.
- ✓ Inhale as you look up and let your stomach drop down toward the mat.
- ✓ Exhale as you tuck your chin into your chest, draw your navel toward your spine, and arch your spine toward the ceiling.
- ✓ Maintain awareness of your body as you do this movement.
- ✓ Focus on noting and releasing tension in your body.
- ✓ Continue this fluid movement for at least 1 minute.

2. Downward-Facing Dog

This traditional forward bend can be restful and rejuvenating. Practicing this pose can help relieve back pain and sciatica. It helps to work out imbalances in the body and improves strength.

Muscles worked:

- ✓ Hamstrings
- ✓ Deltoids
- ✓ Gluteus Maximus
- ✓ Triceps
- ✓ Quadriceps

To do this:

- ✓ Get on all fours.
- ✓ Place your hands in alignment under your wrists and your knees under your hips.
- ✓ Press into your hands, tuck your toes under, and lift up your knees.
- ✓ Bring your sitting bones up toward the ceiling.

✓ Keep a slight bend in your knees and lengthen your spine and tailbone.

✓ Keep your heels slightly off the ground.

✓ Press firmly into your hands.

✓ Distribute your weight evenly between both sides of your body, paying attention to the position of your hips and shoulders.

✓ Keep your head in line with your upper arms or with your chin tucked in slightly.

✓ Hold this pose for up to 1 minute.

3. Extended Triangle

This classic standing posture may help alleviate backache, sciatica, and neck pain. It stretches your spine, hips, and groin, and strengthens your shoulders, chest, and legs. It may also help relieve stress and anxiety.

Muscles worked:

✓ Latissimus Dorsi

✓ Internal Oblique

- ✓ Gluteus Maximus And Medius
- ✓ Hamstrings
- ✓ Quadriceps

To do this:

- ✓ From standing, walk your feet about 4 feet apart.
- ✓ Turn your right toes to face forward, and your left toes out at an angle.
- ✓ Lift your arms parallel to the floor with your palms facing down.
- ✓ Tilt forward and hinge at your right hip to come forward with your arm and torso.
- ✓ Bring your hand to your leg, a yoga block, or onto the floor.
- ✓ Extend your left arm up toward the ceiling.
- ✓ Look up, forward, or down.
- ✓ Hold this pose for up to 1 minute.
- ✓ Repeat on the opposite side.

4. Sphinx Pose

This gentle backbend strengthens your spine and buttocks. It stretches your chest, shoulders, and abdomen. It may also help relieve stress.

Muscles worked:

- ✓ Erector Spinae
- ✓ Gluteal Muscles
- ✓ Pectoralis Major
- ✓ Trapezius
- ✓ Latissimus Dorsi

To do this:

- ✓ Lie on your stomach with your legs extended behind you.
- ✓ Engage the muscles of your lower back, buttocks, and thighs.
- ✓ Bring your elbows under your shoulders with your forearms on the floor and your palms facing down.
- ✓ Slowly lift up your upper torso and head.

✓ Gently lift and engage your lower abdominals to support your back.

✓ Ensure that you're lifting up through your spine and out through the crown of your head, instead of collapsing into your lower back.

✓ Keep your gaze straight ahead as you fully relax in this pose, while at the same time remaining active and engaged.

✓ Stay in this pose for up to 5 minutes.

5. Cobra Pose

This gentle backbend stretches your abdomen, chest, and shoulders. Practicing this pose strengthens your spine and may soothe sciatica. It may also help to relieve stress and fatigue that can accompany back pain.

Muscles worked:

✓ Hamstrings

✓ Gluteus Maximus

- ✓ Deltoids
- ✓ Triceps
- ✓ Serratus Anterior

To do this:

- ✓ Lie on your stomach with your hands under your shoulders and your fingers facing forward.
- ✓ Draw your arms in tightly to your chest. Don't allow your elbows to go out to the side.
- ✓ Press into your hands to slowly lift your head, chest, and shoulders.
- ✓ You can lift partway, halfway, or all the way up.
- ✓ Maintain a slight bend in your elbows.
- ✓ You can let your head drop back to deepen the pose.
- ✓ Release back down to your mat on an exhale.

✓ Bring your arms by your side and rest your head.

✓ Slowly move your hips from side to side to release tension from your lower back.

6. Locust Pose

This gentle backbend may help relieve lower back pain and fatigue. It strengthens the back torso, arms, and legs.

Muscles worked:

✓ Trapezius

✓ Erector Spinae

✓ Gluteus Maximus

✓ Triceps

To do this:

✓ Lie on your stomach with your arms next to your torso and your palms facing up.

✓ Touch your big toes together and turn out your heels to the side.

- ✓ Place your forehead lightly on the floor.
- ✓ Slowly lift your head, chest, and arms partway, halfway, or all the way up.
- ✓ You may bring your hands together and interlace your fingers behind your back.
- ✓ To deepen the pose, lift your legs.
- ✓ Look straight ahead or slightly upward as you lengthen the back of your neck.
- ✓ Remain in this pose for up to 1 minute.
- ✓ Rest before repeating the pose.

7. Bridge Pose

This is a backbend and inversion that can be stimulating or restorative. It stretches the spine and it may relieve backaches and headaches.

Muscles worked:

- ✓ Rectus And Transverse Abdominis
- ✓ Gluteus Muscles
- ✓ Erector Spinae
- ✓ Hamstrings

To do this:

- ✓ Lie on your back with your knees bent and heels drawn into your sitting bones.
- ✓ Rest your arms alongside your body.
- ✓ Press your feet and arms into the floor as you lift your tailbone up.
- ✓ Continue lifting until your thighs are parallel to the floor.
- ✓ Leave your arms as they are, bringing your palms together with interlaced fingers under your hips, or placing your hands under your hips for support.
- ✓ Hold this pose for up to 1 minute.
- ✓ Release by slowly rolling your spine back down to the floor, vertebra by vertebra.
- ✓ Drop your knees in together.
- ✓ Relax and breathe deeply in this position.

8. Half Lord of the Fishes

This twisting pose energizes your spine and helps to relieve backache. It stretches your hips, shoulders, and neck. This pose can help alleviate fatigue and stimulate your internal organs.

Muscles worked:

- ✓ rhomboids
- ✓ serratus anterior
- ✓ erector spinae
- ✓ pectoralis major
- ✓ psoas
- ✓ To do this:
- ✓ From a seated position, draw your right foot in close to your body.
- ✓ Bring your left foot to the outside of your leg.
- ✓ Lengthen your spine as you twist your body to the left.
- ✓ Take your left hand to the floor behind you for support.
- ✓ Move your right upper arm to the outside of your left thigh, or wrap your elbow around your left knee.

✓ Try to keep your hips square to deepen the twist in your spine.

✓ Turn your gaze to look over either shoulder.

✓ Hold this pose for up to 1 minute.

✓ Repeat on the other side.

9. Two-Knee Spinal Twist

This restorative twist promotes movement and mobility in the spine and back. It stretches your spine, back, and shoulders. Practicing this pose can help relieve pain and stiffness in your back and hips.

Muscles worked:

✓ Erector Spinae

✓ Rectus Abdominis

✓ Trapezius

✓ Pectoralis Major

To do this:

- ✓ Lie on your back with your knees drawn into your chest and your arms extended to the side.
- ✓ Slowly lower your legs to the left side while keeping your knees as close together as possible.
- ✓ You may place a pillow under both knees or in between your knees.
- ✓ You can use your left hand to gently press down on your knees.
- ✓ Keep your neck straight, or turn it to either side.
- ✓ Focus on breathing deeply in this position.
- ✓ Hold this pose for at least 30 seconds.
- ✓ Repeat on the opposite side.

10. Child's Pose

This gentle forward fold is the perfect way to relax and release tension in your neck and back. Your spine is lengthened and stretched. Child's Pose also stretches your hips, thighs, and ankles. Practicing this pose can help relieve stress and fatigue.

Muscles Worked:

- ✓ Gluteus Maximus
- ✓ Rotator Cuff Muscles
- ✓ Hamstrings
- ✓ Spinal Extensors

To do this:

- ✓ Sit back on your heels with your knees together.
- ✓ You can use a bolster or blanket under your thighs, torso, or forehead for support.
- ✓ Bend forward and walk your hands in front of you.
- ✓ Rest your forehead gently on the floor.
- ✓ Keep your arms extended in front of you or bring your arms alongside your body with your palms facing up.

✓ Focus on releasing tension in your back as your upper body falls heavy into your knees.

✓ Remain in this pose for up to 5 minutes.

Does it really work?

One small study assessed the effects of either yoga practice or physical therapy over the course of one year. The participants had chronic back pain and showed similar improvement in pain and activity limitation. Both groups were less likely to use pain medications after three months. Separate research found that people who practiced yoga showed small to moderate decreases in pain intensity in the short term.

Practice was also found to slightly increase participants' short- and long-term function.

Chair yoga can be useful for older adults who have difficulty with balance or want to improve their strength while minimizing the risk of falls. Chairs can provide stability or make an exercise easier for a beginner. People can do chair yoga with the help of a physical therapist or yoga instructor or by following tutorials they might find online or in a book.

The movements typically involve sitting in the chair while stretching and holding poses or standing and using the chair for balance.

Does chair yoga really work?

Yes — the research to date on chair yoga for older adults is positive. However, the studies so far have tended to involve a low number of participants. Chair yoga may:

Improve strength: A small study of 35 older women in community care found that 12 weeks of chair yoga improved strength in the hands, arms, and legs. However, this study was small, so more research is necessary.

Improve balance: The same study also found improvements in balance, agility, gait, and limb flexibility following chair yoga.

Help those with arthritis: A 2023 study of 85 Taiwanese women with knee osteoarthritis (OA) found that regular chair yoga improved functional fitness, suggesting it could be helpful for people with joint conditions.

Reduce joint pain: Another study from 2016 of older adults with OA found that an 8-week chair yoga program reduced joint pain. This effect remained for at least 3 months after the program finished.

Reduce the fear of falls: A small 2012 study of older adults with a median age of 88 years found that 8 weeks of regular chair yoga may improve mobility and decrease the fear of falls among this age group, with no adverse effects. However, this study had a very low number of participants, so more research is needed.

There is also significant evidence that yoga more generally improves the quality of life in older adults. A 2019 systematic reviewTrusted Source of previous studies found that this form of exercise can benefit physical strength and flexibility, as well as mental well-being, in this age group.

Is it ever too late to start yoga?

It is never too late to start yoga. Some of the benefits can begin from the first session. Even if a person cannot manage much exercise initially, making gradual steps toward better strength and balance can lead to rewards over time. However, if a person has difficulty with certain movements, or they are not seeing any results, they may benefit from speaking with a physical therapist or yoga instructor who has experience working with older adults.

If a person has difficulty exercising due to pain, injury, unexplained fatigue, or muscle weakness, they should speak with a doctor before trying any new form of exercise.

Chair Yoga Poses for Older Adults

Below are some chair yoga poses. To start, a person will need a stable chair without arms. It should not have wheels or castors. Wear comfortable clothing that allows for stretching. Additional tools, such as yoga blocks or a rolled-up towel, can also be useful, but they are not essential. If any movement feels painful, stop and speak with a doctor.

1. **Upward Salute Pose**

To try this pose:

- ✓ Sit in the chair, with the back straight and feet planted on the floor, parallel and hip-width apart.
- ✓ Inhaling, raise both arms toward the ceiling. Keep the shoulders relaxed and the back straight, without arching.
- ✓ Exhale while lowering the arms.
- ✓ Seated Mountain Pose

To do this pose:

- ✓ Sit in a chair and bring the soles of the feet to the floor.
- ✓ Align the ankles and knees.
- ✓ Elongate the spine from bottom to top, extending the vertebrae.
- ✓ Inhale while drawing the shoulders forward and up.
- ✓ Exhale while rolling the shoulders down and back.
- ✓ Repeat as desired.

2. Seated Cat-Cow Pose

To do this pose:

- ✓ Sit in a stable chair, with the back straight and feet planted on the floor.
- ✓ Bring the hands onto the knees.
- ✓ While inhaling, lift the chest and move the shoulders back, looking upward.
- ✓ Exhale while rounding the back, bringing the chin toward the body.
- ✓ Repeat as desired.

3. Seated Pigeon Pose

To do this pose:

- ✓ Sit upright on the chair, with the feet on the floor.
- ✓ Bring the right ankle up onto the left thigh, keeping the right knee and ankle aligned.
- ✓ Hold the pose for a few seconds. To stretch more, bend forward from the hips.
- ✓ Repeat on the other side.

4. Downward-Facing Dog with chair

To try this pose:

- ✓ Stand in front of a chair, with the feet hip-distance apart.
- ✓ Bending from the hips, place the hands on the seat of the chair or grip the sides. Keep the back straight.
- ✓ Step the feet back until the arms are fully extended. Try to keep the heels planted on the ground. If this is difficult, try using a wedge or rolled-up towel to support the heels, or bend the knees.
- ✓ Hold the pose for as long as it feels comfortable.
- ✓ To finish, step the feet forward again and raise the upper body to a standing position.

How often should you do chair yoga?

There is no strict rule about how often people should do chair yoga. The right frequency may depend on a person's current level of fitness, their goals, and how much exercise they can do before they tire. A person may find it beneficial to start with a small amount of chair yoga and then work up to two or three sessions per week. Alternatively, if they can, they can ask a physical therapist what amount is right for them.

Are there any risks?

As with any form of exercise, there are some potential risks when it comes to chair yoga. Even though the risk of falling to the floor is lessened when doing seated poses, there is still a possibility this could happen. It is important to use a very stable chair. Injury is also possible if a person overexerts themselves or strains a muscle.

CONCLUSION

Using a chair doesn't mean your yoga practice will be easier. You can challenge yourself in almost any pose by adding in this handy prop. Now that you see how it can work, you can explore deepening your experience in some of your favorite poses. And if you're sitting in a chair reading this right now, you can begin to turn the time you sit at a desk into part of your fitness routine.

Although recent research supports yoga practice as a way to treat back pain, it may not be appropriate for everyone. Be sure to talk with your doctor before starting any new yoga or exercise program. Yoga provides many benefits for physical and mental health, including relieving stress and anxiety and enhancing mood and sleep quality. If you are unsure how to perform any of these movements, ask a certified yoga instructor for guidance.

They can help you identify any possible risks and help monitor your progress. You can start a home practice with as little as 10 minutes per day. You can use books, articles, and online classes to guide your practice. Once you learn the basics, you can intuitively create your own sessions. If you prefer more hands-on learning, you may wish to take classes at a studio. Be sure to seek out classes and teachers who can cater to your specific needs.

Though the research is hopeful, further studies are needed to confirm and expand upon these findings.

9 798329 857924